Vagus Nerve Stimulation

The Secrets to Activate Your Vagal Tone With 13 Proven Exercises and Methods to Overcome Depression, Relieve Chronic Stress, End Anxiety, and More.

By

Martin Norris

Disclaimer

This publication is designed to provide reliable information on the subject matter only for educational purposes, and it is not intended to provide medical advice for any medical treatment. You should always consult your doctor or physician for guidance before you stop, start, or alter any prescription medications or attempt to implement the methods discussed. This book is published independently by the author and has no affiliation with any brands or products mentioned within it. The author hereby disclaims any responsibility or liability whatsoever that is incurred from the use or application of the contents of this publication by the purchaser or reader. The purchaser or reader is hereby responsible for his or her own actions.

Table of Contents

Introduction

Our world today comes with several kinds of health conditions and problems, such as chronic stress, anxiety, depression, and chronic inflammation, among others. It is no surprise that these conditions are more than likely associated with the malfunctioning of the vagus nerve. This is so because the vagus nerve plays a very important role in the human body, with connections to virtually almost all organs of the human body – relaying signals between the brain and the human organs. Its connection runs from the brain down to the neck, chest, and abdomen. This nerve is responsible for automating the processes related to heart rate, breathing, food digestion, and a lot more. This nerve, which also controls the release of antidepressants and hormones, explains why it impacts virtually every emotional and physiological state we experience, and this includes stress, anxiety, and depression. Should any damage be done to this critical nerve, the consequences can be far too alarming to grasp. Hence, the importance that this nerve is adequately tendered and stimulated for optimal functioning.

To live a healthy life, we must understand how this nerve operates and how we can optimize its operation. To do this, we stimulate the vagus nerve. The stimulation of the vagus nerve can be done in several ways.

This book seeks to educate you on all you need to know about the vagus nerve, its operations, health conditions associated with it, habits, and substances that can impair the functioning of this nerve, and ultimately how you can effectively stimulate the vagus nerve to serve you better. It is not enough to know how to stimulate the vagus nerve, but also what you must do to ensure it does not malfunction and lead to health complications.

So if you are ready, then lets jump right into it, shall we?

Chapter 1

Getting to Know Your Vagus Nerve

What is the Vagus Nerve?

The human body is made up of various parts, contributing their individual roles to the general well being of the body. Each of these distinct parts are a collection of various nerves, tissues, cells and systems. The complex nature of the body, as studied by some, has continued to be a wonder that truly amazes medical experts.

The nervous system is the most complex of all systems whose role cannot be overlooked. It is the system in the body that controls the transmission of information and nerve impulses from one part of the body to another. Think of it as a car with different wiring connections running through every single part of it. When a task is about to be carried out, these wires send signals to the part of the car responsible for that task before initiation can take place. This is how the nervous system functions. No human activity can be carried out in the body without the intervention of the nervous system.

As far as each organ is from each other, the nervous system collectively functions to bring cellular information regarding the task to be carried out.

The nervous system is further divided into the central nervous system and the peripheral nervous system. The central nervous system is made up essentially of the brain and the spinal cord. The peripheral nervous system refers to parts of the nervous system outside the brain and spinal cord. It includes the cranial nerves, spinal nerves, roots and branches, peripheral nerves, and neuromuscular junctions.

When the human body goes to sleep, there are lots of activities that go on to maintain the balance of health and make sure the body remains in a state of rest. You might be tempted to think that the entire body goes on vacation, but no, some organs and systems still have their roles irrespective of what state the body is in. These parts of the body are most likely controlled by the parasympathetic nervous system, which has no definite time of action. They are always active to ensure that the body performs its roles in a steady manner. Functions like digestion, heart rate, regulation of breathing are all brought about by the action of this part of the nervous system.

The vagus nerve is the tenth cranial nerve of the peripheral nervous system. It is a mixed nerve, which means it has both motor and sensory functions. It is a primary component of the parasympathetic nervous system making the roles it performs very essential even to the central nervous system. The ability to carry out specific tasks is attributed to its ability to exert an influence over the entire body through what we call chemoreceptors. The vagus nerve is comprised of different fibers working hand in hand to bring balance in the body. These fibers are classified as sensory and motor fibers. Some may call it afferent and efferent. What this means is that these fibers are capable of conveying both motor and sensory signals from the various organs of the body to the brain where the information is interpreted and the next line of action taken coherently.

Anatomy of the Vagus Nerve

The vagus nerve is the longest cranial nerve in the body. It derives its name from the wandering nature and complex branching into different areas of the body. This branching is not only restricted to the brain and the neck but also extends to the abdomen, lungs and heart. It is the tenth pair of nerves which leaves the brain. To help us know more about its roles and operations, we need to take a critical look at its anatomy.

From the Brain

The vagus nerve is found to take its origin in the medulla oblongata of the brain. The vagus nerve comprises of four nuclei whose axons emanate from or converge in the brain. These nuclei are known as the dorsal motor nucleus, the nucleus ambiguous, the solitary nucleus and the spinal trigeminal nucleus. These distinct connection have their various functions in the intestinal tract, lungs, mouth, throat, even as far as the heart. The vagus nerve travels out of the brain through the jugular foramen, where it is joined by an accessory nerve leading into the neck.

Down to the Neck

The main trunk of the vagus nerve is bound by the trachea and esophagus and on the lateral side, the carotid artery and a jugular vein located by it. The right part of the nerve branching from the vagus nerve has its base at the neck and travels under the subclavian artery. It then takes an upward movement into the larynx. The left part of the nerve has a similar route it takes but loops around the ligamentum arteriosus. This movement still continues into parts of the thorax.

Down to the Thorax

The vagus nerve forms a trunk when viewed from the right and another trunk at the left. The branching of the various trunks is what constitutes the formation of the esophagus muscles. These muscles aid the smooth passage of food particles down it. Other branches that arise from the thorax include the left laryngeal nerve. This takes its root at the aorta of the heart before ascending into a collection of muscles of the larynx. We also have the cardiac branches which regulate heart rate and provide sensations necessary for the organ. An opening in the diaphragm helps the vagus nerve gain entrance into the abdomen.

Down to the Abdomen

The vagal branching emanating from the thorax gains entrance through a diaphragmatic opening into the areas of the abdomen, where it further divides into branches that supply the esophagus, small and large intestine. These are all connected to enable it to gain control over digestive operations. The vagus nerve connections in the abdomen are so designed to aid the smooth transition of food particles from one part of the intestines to the other. Some key information is being transferred to ensure complete regulation of digestive activities from the brain. As earlier stated, the brain functions by sending and receiving impulses that are connected to the various body organs.

Why is the Vagus Nerve So Important?

The vagus nerve plays several roles in keeping the body functioning at an optimum level. Some of its functions are;

Swallowing of Food

Swallowing of food is one of the most crucial activities your body undertakes. This activity is very crucial both to your health and stability as food digestion begins here. Digestion is possible because food is being taken down the mouth into the various body organs where it is processed. The movement of the food through the esophagus is aided by the transmissions of the vagus nerve. The vagus nerve helps control the coherent movement of food as well as breathing. While food is being swallowed, the air passage is paused so as to avoid choking. The smooth transition of the muscles helps the food to be pushed down to the esophagus, where procession continues.

Digestion of Food

The digestion of food is brought about by the contraction and relaxation of your stomach muscles. This contraction enables the food to be pushed down into the intestines. The vagus nerve essentially aids this movement by ensuring that nerve signals are sent from the brain to the stomach muscles so that the vibrations and movement can begin. Imagine what will happen if your brain is unaware that digestion should take place. What this means is that the food swallowed will remain in the stomach dormant for a long period of time, which results in various health implications.

Fighting Inflammation

The vagus nerve is responsible for sending impulses that prevent inflammation of body organs. Inflammations are temporary and brief occurrences resulting from the inability of the immune system to restore a balance in the homeostasis and metabolism in the body. When it happens, the vagus nerve is supposed to send impulses down to the immune defense system to begin secretions of anti-inflammatory chemicals that should be able to work effectively on such inflammations. When this immune response is hindered, there could be further complications that give birth to chronic conditions. For effective immune communication, information must be sent from the brain through the vagus nerve connections so that the inflammations can be addressed immediately its formation begins.

Controls Heart Rate and Blood Pressure

Moderations must be kept in check for any activity the body undertakes, no matter the size and duration. Heart rate and blood pressure regulation are one of those activities that must be under critical regulation to avoid medical complications. When heart rate becomes excessively too fast, there is a loss in the consciousness of the individual and it could cause damages to the heart. The heart functions by contraction and relaxation of muscles. These muscles must be put under an appropriate check to make sure it doesn't exceed a stipulated pressure. Blood flow is also associated with heart rate. When the heart rate is slow or fast, it has a direct effect on the pressure with which the blood is pushed out into different areas of the body. The vagus nerve is responsible for the control of these activities.

Facilitates Breathing

The communication that ensues between the vagus nerve and the diaphragm is what aids smooth breathing processes. Breathing is another involuntary activity that isn't brought to a pause whether the individual is awake or not. Breathing processes are what bring the supply of oxygen into the body and without this, important activities cannot be undertaken. The movement of air through the lungs and diaphragmatic muscle movements are controlled by the vagus nerve. Since breathing has to be controlled by the brain, the vagus nerve sends information down to the various organs concerned so that they can carry out their designed functions.

Provides Ear Sensations

The sensations experienced by the ear are brought about by the transmissions of impulses through the vagus nerve. This communication can be used to modify hearing. Scientific research shows that pairing the vagus nerve system with produced tones increases the plasticity of sound. This is brought to effect by the activation of certain neuromodulators in the brain. This release, when paired up with the presentation of sound coming from the ear, sends back a plastic reflection of sound waves throughout the entire auditory system. The sensations associated with the ear are on account of the sound waves that it comes in contact with. This sensation must be interpreted by the brain for better understanding.

Managing Hunger and Satiety

The vagus nerve is responsible for the feeling of hunger and satisfaction. The communication that brings about the sensation of hunger and the satisfaction that comes with food intake takes place along the vagus nerve. When food is consumed by the body and proper digestion has taken place, the stomach sends signals through the vagus nerve to the brain so that eating processes can be brought to a halt. No matter how hungry you might get, there is always a stipulated amount of food your body can take. This moderation is what prevents overfeeding and the complications that are associated with such. When the body is also in short supply of food, it also sends back information to your brain to alert the need to begin food intake. This desire is what creates the need for the selection of food types to be consumed. When this information reaches your brain, it is being interpreted so that the reason for the food can be accompanied. For example, you might have expended so much energy and now, in need of energy-giving food, your brain will opt for the intake of carbohydrate-rich food.

Gut-Brain Communication

Your gut and brain are connected together through the vagus nerve. This connection influences the brain by determining the impulses being sent across throughout the body. Neurotransmitters are what produce the different feelings that are associated with the body. They are generated in the brain and being passed down to the various organs where they are to be felt. If you've ever had any feeling ranging from excitement, sorrow, pain, they are all associated with the gut-brain communication brought about through the vagus nerve. These chemical secretions aren't controlled by conscious efforts but are part of the subconscious activities the brain regulates.

Chapter 2

Vagal Tone and Why It Matters

Vagal tone is an important body parameter. This is because of the significance of the vagal nerve to the body. Essential body functions that are automated and isolated from conscious control are all moderated by the vagal nerve. For optimal healthy performance, the vagal nerve must be in good condition. Vagal tone is used to determine the state of the vagal nerve. It tells us the present condition of the vagal nerve and helps us identify the effects that would be associated with such manifestation. From numerous research, scientists have been able to come up with effective ways of distinguishing the common types of vagal tone the body experiences. The classification modes are the high vagal tone and low vagal tone.

High Vagal Tone

The increase in the vagal tone of the body has been identified as a good phenomenon. Good in the sense that so many body functions are carried out optimally when the vagal tone is high. Since the vagal nerve is one of the most important cranial nerves and, in fact, the most complicated, its significance is too much to neglect.

Many people complain of difficulties having their blood regulated and distributed effectively around the body. This challenge is associated with low vagal tone. When the vagal tone of an individual is relatively high, you can be rest assured that he/she would have better blood and sugar regulation. Blood regulation, which includes blood pressure, and heart rate, is essential for the body to remain in its state of equilibrium. The rate at which blood leaves the heart into other areas of the body is what determines the ability of the heart to carry out its basic procedures.

With the emergence of better blood distribution, heart complications like strokes are avoided. Stroke is a medical condition arising from the inability of the blood to get to certain areas of the body. Stroke is not limited to any part of the body as any shortage of blood flow will eventually bring about this disease condition. High vagal tone is also accompanied with better digestion as enzymes that control the digestive processes are most readily released due to the communication between the stomach and the brain. Without the communication of this information with the brain on the type of food to be broken down, the brain cannot prescribe the appropriate enzyme to be produced. The inability of the body to engage in proper digestion only bring about complications and medical consequences. Another important aspect of having a high vagal tone is the ability of an individual to have a better mood and less anxious emotions. This, on its own, is a stress relief that helps the body in dealing with stress.

Low Vagal Tone

The decrease in the value of measured vagal time can be said to have its effects on various body operations. As much as this needs to be avoided, we must first understand its implications to the human body. Not many are aware of the dangers that are connected with having a low vagal tone. This is why they have paid little or/no attention to know what the state of their vagal tone is.

One of the dangers of having a low vagal tone is cardiovascular conditions. These conditions are associated with the heart. The heart is a very delicate organ and must be treated with care. The neurons and control mechanisms that automate activities must ensure that it functions at optimum capacity. Heart conditions may result from the inability of the blood being pumped to be circulated around the entire body creating room for the decay of some organs or death of cells.

Another implication of a low vagal tone is depression. This has been at the peak of emotional disorders and conditions facing today's world. You have lots of young and aged people going into depression of varying degrees. Some have attributed it to some spiritual or mystic event. They are still ignorant that feelings and emotions are impulses that are sent from the brain. The inability of the vagus nerve to pick up these signals or picking at reduced speed can bring an individual into a state of depression. Depression can be triggered by a lot of factors, both psychological or physiological. When depressive moods begin to set in, it is the duty of the vagus nerve to release anti depressing hormones to counteract the reaction.

Chronic fatigue syndrome is another associated phenomenon with low vagal tone. This arises from the continued tiredness experienced by the body, even when it shouldn't. This will make an individual feel weak most of the time and induce lesser productivity. People with this kind of condition have difficulties carrying out predefined tasks and objectives. They are not in control of when the feeling of tiredness would set in. They are only accustomed to the feelings when it fully manifests.

People with low vagal tone should also be prepared to face serious inflammatory conditions. These arise from the inability of the immune system to secret anti-inflammatory antigens to defend the body. This especially can bring about different types of health conditions like bowel diseases, arthritis and so many others. The brain's inability to send information to the immune system to begin deployment of antibodies will further complicate the situation on the ground. It is advisable to perform regular checkups to avoid your vagal tone from depreciating that much.

Measuring Your Vagal Tone

The measurement of the vagal tone comes with a scientific method. A common method being applied today is the heart rate count during breathing. When you take in air and breathe out the waste, there is always a rhythm and rate at which your heart produces. This heart rate speeds up a little when air is being taken into the body. It is slower when exhalation takes place. The difference in the heart rate between inhalation and exhalation gives an idea of how low or high the vagal tone is.

What is Heart Rate Variability

Heart rate variability is simply the measure of the difference between two successive heartbeats. As stated previously, the heart is controlled by the autonomic nervous system. This helps the activity to keep going whether the body is awake or not. The optimum functioning of the heartbeat at times when the body is resting is so that the body cells don't die due to shortages in blood and oxygen. The red blood cells are what carry the oxygen to the distinct parts of the body. The regulation of the heart rate isn't controlled by your conscious desire to do so. It is already built into your brain system to exert a great amount of influence on the heart rate. Have you imagined why your heartbeat tends to go up faster when you have increased brain activity? It is because your brain activity has been set to have a direct effect on the heart and rate of blood flow.

The same way breathing, digestion are being controlled and automated, that is the same way heart functions are regulated. The autonomic nervous system can also be subdivided into the sympathetic and parasympathetic, respectively. The parasympathetic components can be tagged as the flight and response mechanism. This part of the nervous system is what gives you the urge to take action when an activity threatens the state of safety.

The brain works like a computer, carrying out diverse kinds of information processing. Through the help of the autonomic nervous system, signals are being sent to various parts of the body to trigger the implementation of various activities. This response is not limited to a bad day at the office, or when a piece of exciting news is mentioned, with our bodies having different ways of dealing with shock or when excited. This is accompanied by a spike or reduction in the rate at which blood is being pumped. The balance of this response and trigger can be taken off with a balance on things like a healthy diet, relationships, and exercise.

Why Check Heart Rate Variability?

Heart rate variability is a very good tool for the identification of imbalances that are associated with the autonomic nervous system. The ability of an individual to switch moods from one to another is a good reason for this analysis. The heartbeat when a person is in his/her flight mode is always high. This can be used to test for the health of the vagal tone. The speed with which an individual can switch modes is attributed to the health of his autonomous nervous system. Research over the years has brought to light the relationship between low heart rate variability and increasing depression cases. This can be a source of deaths emanating from heart diseases.

Higher heart rate variability will help the individual maintain better cardiovascular conditions and create a defense system against the effect of stress. It can also be used to determine the kind of lifestyle being lived and can help with improving one's way of living. HRV has also been said to have a transforming effect on the physical attributes of the individual, which might include sleep, mindfulness, meditation and the rest. You can now be sure that your nervous system is still on track and free from the influence of emotions, thoughts and feelings.

Interpreting Heart Rate Variability Results

One thing to note is that heart rate is one essential metric value whose determination lies not just on the speed of blood being pumped but on the timely variations that spike with each heartbeat. It has been already seen that individuals with higher HRV (heart rate variability) result come out having better health when compared to individuals with lower HRV. This is so because their hearts are more active, thus increasing the ability of the heart to take more desired volumes of blood to the different parts of the body when needed. This activity can also be seen as a means of disease prevention. It is being said that as blood flows through the blood veins, it takes along with it the contamination that would have constituted ill health.

This is true for many reasons; one of them being that persons with increased blood activity either through daily exercise or muscle activity have reduced risks of falling ill. This can be well seen in athletics and sportsmen. For the human body to remain in healthy conditions, blood flow accompanied by a good heart rate should be maintained. A low heart rate variability result gives rise to the formation of many killer disease conditions. Having low HRV doesn't necessarily mean that the disease condition has been formed yet, but with time the strength of the body in fighting against most of these infections would be reduced.

HRV data isn't just significant to heart conditions alone. It can also be used to reduce emotional, mental and behavioral patterns. Studies have shown that the emotional state of an individual has a direct relationship in the results of an HRV test. For example, a man who just came back from his office, where he just received a promotion would have a happy and excited emotional state. This state of excitement would give birth to a high HRV value. This can be characterized by reduced cause for worry, less formation of disease conditions and so on.

Medical experts have informed us that the more a man stays happy, the healthier he tends to become. This emanated from the series of experiments carried out on various calibers of individuals. The results came out with those having better minds and happy emotions living above the expected medical threshold. Worries, anxiety and fear are all sources of health drains. The time spent thinking and worrying about the state of things could be invested in making the most of life. You can even discover that your most productive moments come at times when you are better relaxed, happy and in no sad emotional state. Thoughts and ideas seem to flow perfectly, reducing the risks of brain fatigue.

Another revelation by research has been the dependence of HRV values on other factors like self-control. Self-control arises from the ability of the individual to be self-aware of himself. His control over his entire body comes from his ability to take control of his mental activities. Putting to check the thoughts he allows into his mind exercise control of his entire body and mental activity.

The stress that comes with rigorous brain activity can be filtered to a large extent. Self-control is of a deliberate act, where you try to possess conscious power over your mind and life. Most motivational speakers challenge you to take control of your life by charting the way forward through ideas and innovations. This cannot be possible when you have lots of things to worry about. Editing this time and energy wasters will give you the required energy to break past your limitations.

Stress management, as advised by many, is better achieved when individuals pay attention to managing all that comes to reduce or abnormally increase the heart rate. Though heart rate should be moderately high, it doesn't permit for excessively high heart rates. The higher the heart rate above normal, the more dreadful it becomes. Many with good social skills have been traced back to healthy emotional and heart conditions. The happiness an individual exhibits can be transmitted to all those around, thus helping him connect better with people. You can now see that the applications of heart rate variability give beyond just medical examination and benefits but also into the social world. Imagine the fact that a good HRV value could just be the reason why you get the next promotion at the office due to increased productivity and efficient service delivery. It could also be the reason why your relationship issues with those around you gets resolved.

The arousal for the tendencies for physiological stress can be well monitored through HRV tests. This can predict and show you the occurrences of a low heart rate variability value. The awareness of this result will guide you in making healthier choices that will eliminate the challenges that come with such. Investigation can be carried out through varying methods.

These methods can include the ECG (Electrocardiogram) devices.

When we try to analyze the little differences present in the interval between heartbeats, we attempt to trace the signals that create the heart heat to the sources where they are coming from. This could be the SNS (Sympathetic Nervous System) or PNS (Parasympathetic Nervous System). The PNS and SNS are collectively responsible for making and establishing the heartbeats. Knowing the body system that is active will give the necessary information on the level of stress received by the body and how well it copes under pressure.

There are two known methods for analyzing heart rate variability. They are the time domain and the frequency domain analysis. In both methods, the interval between heartbeats is measured. This could also be called the RR- intervals.

Time-domain analysis

The time-domain analysis tells how the HRV tends to change as time progresses. It can also be used to estimate the sympathetic and parasympathetic activity. Among the many domain characters used are RR, SDNN, TINN, etc.

When grouping, intervals are placed in bands according to their length. An example would be 700-800, 500-600, 800-900 ms. The intervals are then categorized to see how many of them would fall into the bands allocated.

Frequency-Domain Analysis

To be able to identify the process that the body is undergoing, we would carry out a frequency domain analysis. This will tell us if the body is currently undergoing recovery or stress. Knowledge of what process is being carried out will help us know how to manage the conditions and channel energy towards the most productive outcome. For recovery processes, the body is trying to regain lost energy. The heart-pumping rate at this point is quite faster than normal, especially as we apply procedures to increase the heart rate significantly. For stress processes, the body needs to reduce the heart rate significantly.

In the extraction of these parameters, each length of the interval is changed into waves so that the frequencies can be measured. The waves are separated into low and high frequencies and very low-frequency bands.

The analysis of the parameters mentioned will give doctors and health coaches the knowledge of the body's coping mechanism with pressure, the effect of changes like stress, relocation to zero gravity surroundings, and increases in workout loads. The unfortunate thing is that the interpretation of high rate variability data isn't a universal experiment where the values could be generalized for all cases. You can have a varying number of factors that could be at play, which would cause fluctuations of results. An example of such a fracture would be the time at which the individual's nervous system responds more to the stress signals, post HRV measurement results, etc. What could be an indication of high stress for one might, to our surprise, be in a normal range for someone else. This has made us confine HRV to remote fields like space, medicine and sports. This can afford much time and resources for tests to be carried out in one person.

Welltory provides personalized HRV Interpretations without labs tests

A new technology has been developed, which gives more specific interpretation of the HRV. This method utilizes data in automating the processes previously carried out manually. The main advantage over other methods is the vast database comprising over two million HRV measurements already enriched with health and lifestyle data. You can imagine having two million data points to work with, you can be sure of better accuracy.

With this technology, people are separated into four nervous type systems aided through the big data tech. The result of these categories is tested against five thousand already done clinical assessments which have been completed by previous users. This gave birth to the world's first self-learning HRV algorithm capable of adapting to various nervous systems of different individuals. The algorithm developed also accounts for factors like age, gender, the time of the day and even results from past measurements.

To enable an application that is easy to use and well simplified, the standard list of parameters with health scores are replaced with others most easily understood. The scores are accompanied by data driven recommendations, which help people feel better every day. The recommendations can help the individual live a more healthier life free of HRV complications.

The four nervous system classification done by welltory

During a series of studies carried out on heart rate variability, it has been discovered that the heart can be controlled in various ways. In some people, their brain constitutes a major factor in the regulation of their heart rate. In some others, the heart Is self-regulatory. It was discovered that a good number fall in between these categories.

The differences in the regulation carried out with regards to the heart rate variability, further shows how the different number obtained would mean different things for different people. When running the heart rate variability tests, scientists prefer to split people into the different regulation types for proper examination. This classification is carried out through big data technology.

Brain control

This is so supported by subcortical structures that have a huge effect on the functioning of the heart. The subcortical structures cause a simulation of the part of the brain responsible for reflexes, which is essentially constituted in the sympathetic nervous system. The parasympathetic nervous activity of the body is inhibited through the control of reflexes and other lower structures in the brain. The ability of the parasympathetic nervous system to relax is hindered while allowing stimulation of the heart by the sympathetic nervous system. The stimulation can be attributed to two key structures, which are the hypothalamus and the subcortical structures.

Moderate brain control

This is a situation where the hypothalamus assumes control over the regulation of the heart. It is also responsible for triggering reflexes, which in turn stimulate the sympathetic nervous system. These reflexes generated can also bring into active duty, the parasympathetic nervous system depending on what situation is on the ground. For this classification, the sympathetic nervous system never runs inactive. It can be periodically balanced by the functioning of the parasympathetic nervous system.

Moderate auto control

The heart operates autonomously via impulses sent by the sinoatrial node (SA). Its activity is equally modified by the sympathetic and parasympathetic nerves controlled by the brain stem. When the sympathetic and parasympathetic activity is balanced, the heart activity will be well accompanied by an equal number of signals that cause stimulation and relaxation.

Auto control

For this category, the heart operates separately and on its own. It does this through impulses that are sent from the sinoatrial node. The activities that take place here can only be modified by the parasympathetic nervous system. The heart can only receive primarily relaxing signals.

Grouping results obtained from different users

Since there is a wide range of variability values obtained from various users, they can be put under the following categories.

Green — This shows that your heart rate variability value is still within the safe range and your health is still okay.

Red — This tells us that you are currently experiencing one form of stress or another. This stress hasn't reached the threshold to cause notable damages to your body system.

Blue —This gives an idea of the closeness your body gets to its breaking point. The stress being experienced by the body is now taking a high risk of sickness or even damaging body systems.

A baseline is a heart variability range obtained when the individual is calm and okay. This state is predominant in every regulation type. All you have to do is identify when this happens and take a reading of values. For example, two people who fall into the same color zone can still have regulation types different from one another. This will affect how their HRV results change with prevailing circumstances or what is happening to them.

This method of analyzing heart rate variability results has a lot of potentials as it doesn't require expensive equipment and specialized knowledge to undertake. Preventive health care can be more feasible and available to everyone with just the use of a smartphone application. You can now see how convenient and stress-free this process is. You might be having doubts as to if the entire procedure actually works like is explained but yes, it has been tested and proven reliable.

Thousands and good numbers of people have actually used the application to track their health. Through recommendations provided by the application, individuals can be able to recover properly, know what their body needs and providing it. Welltory has become the very first to introduce personalized heart rate variability algorithm, which exposes essential insights about the body's health condition without having to necessarily go through manual processing stages.

Increasing Your Vagal Tone

There are various methods that can be applied to improving the vagal tone. Since there is an increased awareness of the advantages and benefits of having a good vagal tone, the question about how to go about this has risen in different folds. It is one thing to know the importance of something and another to know how to go about it. The methods listed below have a proven result rate, by carefully applying the methods suggested here, you can be rest assured that you would generate higher vagal tones. These methods aren't so sophisticated or scientifically driven so that even the most ignorant individuals can achieve the same results. To be able to improve vagal tone, you need to center your efforts around the parts that have a direct relationship with the vagal nerve. The methods, some of which would be further discussed in the pasges of this book include:

Slow, rhythmic, diaphragmatic breathing

The human body is, by default, trained to breathe from the lungs. This breathing pattern doesn't allow for a more calm and relaxed result. You would notice that most times, when you attempt breathing heavily, your body movement is centered around your chest area.

This signifies that your breathing systems are centered around the lungs and not from the diaphragm. You would need to readjust your system to get used to breathing from your diaphragm. This enables you to maintain slow and rhythmic breathing patterns. This, in turn, helps your vagal nerves become more relaxed and at an appropriate level. This has a direct impact on your heart rate as your heart beats become more organized in the most suitable manner. Better blood diffusion into the different body organs and systems can only be possible when breathing is carried out from the diaphragm. How to perform slow breathing is discussed in subsequent pages of this book.

Humming

Another relaxing technique is the application of humming. Hums come from audible sounds that are made by vibrations on your vocal cords. The biological arrangement of the vocal cords is such in a way that the vagus nerves are connected to them. The importance of this is the fact that vibrations along the vocal cords would automatically trigger the vagus nerve to perform better. As simple as this method seems, it is a very efficient way to trigger the vagus nerve, it is being referred mostly as a mechanical method. While humming, the individual might choose to make use of alphabets or words. Constant practice of this method will ensure an increased vagal tonal result. This is why singers and vocal artists have higher chances of possessing better vocal tones; the frequent vibration of their vocal cords enable such responses. You don't necessarily need to be a musician to achieve the desired result. All you need to do is make sure you consistently keep to the humming routine. Most people prefer to use sentences while humming. It should be noted that there are no specific benchmark on what to hum.

Speaking

Another method that could be used to stimulate the vagus nerve is speaking. Like humming, it has to do with sounds that are generated through the vibration of the vocal cords. Speaking at minimized levels helps keep the vibrations sufficient enough to evoke a response on the vagal nerve. This type of speaking doesn't mean that your voice must be pitched at a certain level. The theory of sound production in the mouth is brought about by the vibration of waves. To eliminate the adverse effect of this method, individuals are advised to mind the number of hours spent on talking. In as much as the procedure can bring tangible results, you should also know that talking is energy-draining/consuming. You should then be mindful of the degree to which you engage this method to avoid adding more stress to the body.

Mediation

This is a very effective tool being deployed in vagal tone increment. To carry this out, the individual is advised to focus his/her thoughts on good memories of himself, acts of love and kindness, and so on. By constantly doing so, the vagus nerve devices more stimulation to function better. A study carried out in 2010 shows that positive emotions have a direct effect on the social engagement of a person, which in turn affects the vagus nerve. Sadness is an emotional condition associated with low vagal tone. Since the motive behind all of this is to increase the vagal tone, anything capable of helping the mind get into an excited state is welcomed. At this point, many neurons are more fired up and ready to transmit signals. The nervous system is said to be at the peak of its performance at this period. You must guard against worries, events and situations that come to induce sadness and sorrow if you must see that your vagal tone doesn't depreciate.

Balancing the gut microbiome

Micro biomes are small bacteria organisms that can be found in the gut tracks. The presence of these microorganisms helps improve the tone of the vagal nerve.

These simple procedures have an implication on the general health of the individual. They have far-reaching positive effects; they include the prevention of inflammations. Inflammations could be very expensive to treat and manage, which makes prevention a better option. Since the application of these exercises ensures, to a large extent, the prevention of inflammation, they should be more encouraged for every person. Other conditions that are also avoided include digestive upsets arising from the inability of the vagus nerve to carry out hormonal indicators for the production of necessary digestive enzymes. You can also prevent high blood pressure-related diseases. Most of these diseases come from the inability of the heart to regulate itself.

Vagal tone exercises are also a recommended preventive action for depression cases. Mediation, which is very helpful to human health, contributes its role to the elevation of the self-esteem of the individual and brings positive thoughts to the mind of the individual. Depression emanates from the lack of belief and trust in one's own self. This would progress to suicidal and low living standards. A good vagal tone can help prevent all these possibilities. Studies have shown that individuals who have low vagal tone end up having more signs of depression than others.

A Short message from the Author:

Hey, I hope you are enjoying the book? I would love to hear your thoughts!

Many readers do not know how hard reviews are to come by and how much they help an author.

I would be incredibly grateful if you could take just 60 seconds to write a short review on the product page of this book from where the purchase was made, even if it is a few sentences!

Thanks for the time taken to share your thoughts!

Chapter 3

Conditions Associated with the Vagus Nerve

Chronic Stress and Anxiety

Stress is the body's default response to any kind of engaging demand, whether social or emotional. Any type of task required to be carried out by the body can be a constituent of stress. This is not limited to just school or office challenges; they could also include events that are traumatic and deeply painful. It could be the loss of a loved one.

It is important to pay attention to the way stress affects your psychological and physiological structure. This will help you come up with ways of dealing with them as they occur irrespective of whether they are major or minor occurrences. Stress can be attributed to a failure in the vagal nerve to perform specific functions. The vagal nerve helps send information to the brain in times of stress so that hormones can be released that would balance these feelings. The inability of this response to come in as fast as required opens up the body to longer-lasting effects of stress in the body. There are certain things to take note of stress and the way it operates. A few of such points are listed below.

1. Stress affects everyone.

Virtually no one is left out of the effects of stress, young, old, sick and healthy. It is one phenomenon that is common to all. As long as your body develops the need to carry out a task, you aren't prohibited from being stressed. There are various types of stress that come with varying consequences, some small while others are greater. Triggers of stress might just have to showcase on a few occasions while others continue repeating themselves over a long period of time. You would find out that some people tend to cope with the stress far better than others because their recovery mechanisms differ.

Examples of stress include:

Pressures from school and academic activities. This comes with lots of health challenges because it has to do with brain-related fatigue. You could also have family and daily responsibilities added to it. At the top of individuals who experience this are the mothers and caregivers. Taking care of a family can be quite exhausting, especially when you have to cope with the inadequacies of others, it is easy to go into a state of stress.

We also have stress brought about by the negative play of events. This kind happens to trigger lots of other reactions. Imagine having to lose someone you dearly loved to the cold arms of death. For some weeks or even months for some individuals, they find it difficult to get over the pain and this will tell on other activities they carry out. You get to see the lack of concentration, anger, sorrow, sadness and bitterness in them. This reduces productivity to a large extent making it Impossible for them to give life their best shot. Some people even go as far as abandoning everything and everyone, taking them into a state of depression and solitude.

Trauma-induced stress is associated with events and experiences such as death, accident, wars, disasters which involve the death and injury of persons either hurt or killed. People who experience this type of stress have frequent emotional and physical symptoms accompanied with it. These symptoms are mild enough to allow for quick recoveries at later times.

2. Not all stress is bad.

You might have the general notion that stress on its own is a bad thing, but no, some stress isn't termed as such. When faced with situations that threaten life, stress signals sent to your brain prepares the body to face the threat. As this happens, your body structure begins to change and enhance in order to be well equipped for the dangers ahead. Your breathing pace increases, muscles become tense, and oxygen usage in the brain spikes up. Sometimes the stress most individuals face spurs them to engage in more opportunities that would reduce such. Take, for example, a man facing serious stress in his workplace; he would take steps to get a new job, which eliminates the stress he is currently facing. Even if it involves him going for an interview or taking some extra certifications, the stress he is currently experiencing has acted as a propellant for a greater achievement.

3. Long-term stress can harm your health.

Long term exposure to stress can be very challenging. This is because in cases like this, the body doesn't receive any signal to return back to normal functioning conditions. The problem starts when the same reactions that would have saved life would also bring reactions that will disable immune, digestive, sleep and reproduction systems. The symptoms that point to this condition are vast, ranging from digestive issues, headache, sleeplessness, sadness, anger and sometimes irritability.

4. There are ways to manage stress.

In order to reduce the impact of stress on the well being of the body, you must take practical steps at minimizing the damage. Stress can be managed and kept at a low-risk rate. There are many tips that can be applied to ensure this, they include.

Being observant: One important key to managing stress is keen observation. This Is because stress manifests in different forms and categories. You must be able to identify the unique pointers that show you are experiencing one form of stress or another. The triggers that give birth to such conditions should also be identified so that you can know how to prevent the occurrence of stress. Some of the signs that you might be experiencing stress could be anger issues, feelings of depression, tiredness, increasing alcohol and drug intake, or difficulties while resting or sleeping.

Talking to a health care provider: Many people overlook the importance of going for regular checkups and medical advice because they think they know how to manage their health. The professionals are there to help you with your health challenges and give advice based on their assessment of the situation. The increase in self-medication has led to the untimely demise of so many people. The effect of stress cannot be adequately determined by just the individual alone; some of them might need professional attention. Stress treatments must be properly recommended by your health officer. Even if you don't know where to begin observation, your consultation with medical practitioners will help guide you into making informed decisions.

Another way you can relieve yourself from stress is by engaging in regular exercises: Allocating a particular number of time for daily exercise contributes a great quota to your physical, mental and emotional health. Taking sequential morning jogs or running exercises can help lighten your mood and relieve you from sad emotions and stress. You could also partake in activities that improve the relaxation of your nerves. There are programs that include meditation, muscle relaxation, breathing exercises that help you achieve relief from stress and anxiety. You should be able to schedule times of your daily routine where you can carry out these exercises.

You can set goals and priorities that help you determine what actions should be carried out at a particular time or the other. This would reduce the weight that comes with having to perform various activities and tasks. You would be doing yourself a great deal by reducing the workload you subject your body to. You would notice that when you have your mind geared towards lots of activities, you tend to get anxious and have so many thoughts in mind that you are unable to meet up with the productivity demanded. Sometimes you need to say no to some tasks if you have already accepted some others. This is a common problem with so many workers. They feel that engaging in different jobs just so that their earnings can increase wouldn't have adverse implications on their health; in the end, they come down with varying degrees of stress.

You need to also stay in touch with others who are currently going through a situation you are facing with stress. They can be a source of emotional and even practical help. By the experiences they share on how they have been able to manage their stress and anxiety situation, you can gain insight on how to manage yours. You need to spend time with friends and family members as a form of relaxation from stress and anxiety. You might be dealing with varying degrees of stress effect, which can be as serious as suicidal thoughts and inclinations to alcohol consumption. Being around the right set of people will help reduce these experiences. Your support group might even include someone who has medical expertise so that he/she can give professional recommendations.

Trauma, PTSD, and Depression

Having to go through ugly experiences like divorce or a loved one shrinking back on his emotional responsibilities to you can trigger negative responses in you. You would be surprised at how much pain you could be induced with on account of the sudden demise of someone you hold close to you. Daily, there are children, teenagers and adults who experience varying degrees of assaults and rape. These events are capable enough to throw them into a state of depression. Today's works are laced with a lot of events and activities that evoke the feeling of trauma and depression. As small as an office place could be, workers and employees have to deal with assaults and traumas of different natures. It is, therefore, important that we pay keen attention to the effect these connote on our day to day life as the vagus nerve is on the front line of these attacks.

Turning on your television, you get to see news about various world climate and environmental disasters. These all can form a string of traumatic responses in an individual.

The imagination that persons have to go through these pains are quite terrible and capable of sending one insane. For most people, they might not display similar sorrow, but trust me, everyone has their breaking point. Constant exposure to these events will definitely take a huge toll on the individual. These piles of traumatic events can lead to depression.

The effect, sometimes of these exposures, is that it can deprive you of your comfort and rest. You would constantly see yourself making frequent flashbacks and recalls of whatever might have taken place. The re-occurrence of traumatic thoughts can be so severe that it takes the individual into a post-traumatic stress disorder state. For others, depression immediately sets in when they hear of these traumatic events that have taken place either to them or others.

A research carried out by a team of scholars reveals that the greatest cause of anxiety and depression in people is traumatic events. This is closely followed by genetically passed mental illnesses. You can now see the huge effects of trauma on persons who are diagnosed with depression and even continuous anxiety.

A person who comes down with depression or anxiety might not know how severe the condition looks until he/she is told. Depression and anxiety are not mere simple conditions. They are very complex since there are no specific triggers or causes that lead to such. They can be generated by the action of various forces and conditions. You can identify the level of stress, anxiety and depression experienced by an individual by analyzing the way their thoughts and steps to come out of such are taken. Most times, people who are deeply consumed in their condition have mostly given up on any form of help or medical attention that can be given to remedy the situation.

Symptoms of Trauma-Induced Depression

Know that when a person experiences an enormous amount of shock beyond what they can normally handle, they are going to gravitate towards trauma. The effect of trauma is mostly felt on the mental and physical well being of the individual. According to statistics, we have classified the various effects of trauma under the following categories. It is important to note that there are more manifestations of trauma than are mentioned here.

- Extreme sadness
- Frequent feeling of sorrow and tears
- Feelings of loss
- Emotional numbness
- Disillusionment
- Loss of appetite
- Difficulties encountered while sleeping
- Resurfacing memories and flashbacks
- Nightmares centered on the event that took place
- Social withdrawal into loneliness

When an individual experiences a traumatic event, it is normal to develop these reactions, but if the duration time where these symptoms persist is more than two weeks, you should begin seeking help. The longer it takes to recover from these events, the more damages caused to the daily life of the individual. The quick recovery of the individual is hinged on the ability of his body to measure up a good vagal tone. Without this, the feelings that are associated with trauma can eat so deep that you begin to think of taking your life. At this point, you don't just need remedial steps, you need to seek professional and medical advice.

Trauma-Induced Depression Treatment

According to studies carried on the body's responses during trauma, it was observed that the body configuration and structure actually changes. With this difference, the effects a person feels when going through traumatic events cannot be easily snapped out of. If you're truly serious about getting over traumatic events, you'll need to talk to some health experts who have experience dealing with such cases. The help you'll obtain will come in three different phases.

Medical intervention

Since depression is the body's way of responding to a trigger, medications, prescribed by a licensed medical practitioner can be administered to bring the chemical imbalance to check.

Therapeutic assistance: You can also be referred to talk to therapeutic experts where you get to share the experiences that caused the trauma and really deal with it once and for all. During these sessions, you will discover that most of the reasons why the experience refused to go away is because you've not talked to someone who can help through words of encouragement.

Peer support: There is a feeling of relief that comes with the knowledge that you have friends and caregivers who are concerned about your well being. The weight of the experiences can be taken off when you come around such persons. They can be a source of encouragement and hope for your downcast state.

You can personally carry out the following steps even as you venture into seeking professional help and advice. They include:

- Spending quality time with friends, family and loved ones

- Engaging in activities you derive joy from

- Exercising regularly

- Practice relaxation techniques

Lack of Social Interaction

This disease condition is characterized by one's inability to relate freely with others. This condition is a true indicator of the poor vagal functioning of the vagal nerve. Several studies have been carried out to determine the role social interaction plays in the health and well being of an individual. When one is healthy mentally, he or she can effectively engage in interactions with the social environment. The social environment comprises of people. Man is naturally a social being, his inability to perform as one is attributed to the poor functioning of the vagal nerve system. This malfunctioning of the vagal nerve initiates the feeling of loneliness and a craving for isolation. The effect of social isolation has been identified as a big risk when it comes to the well being of the individual. In other cases, it even results in death scenarios.

A study made over the years shows that the death experiences experienced by some individuals happened to people with issues in their social network. These persons were either distant from marriages, friends, relatives, and had no obvious membership in notable social organization. They were more prone to more heart conditions and when subjected to accident incidents, they have little or no survival rates. It was also identified that these sets of persons were prone to having stroke and partial paralysis. You can see how devastating being socially isolated can be. You are cut off from the world and love in general. The lack of love, care and support can drive you into insane conditions.

The effects of being lonely have been verified by a series of research and studies. This is not some form of a fairy tale or another. At every stage of a person's life, we can see the effects of social isolation. When questionnaires were varied out on some percentage of people in Finland, it was observed that thirty-nine percent of persons were already suffering from one form of loneliness for some period of time. Five percent of the total percentage were passing through this condition more frequently than others. When a critical examination was done to determine the causes of social isolation, factors like environment (rural or urban), age, level of education, income was reported as likely causes. You would have noticed that when a person begins to feel lesser of himself, he tends to isolate himself from others. He thinks that he shouldn't and can't match up to the social requirement of the people he is supposed to be relating with.

A lot of people are quick to call their inability to relate with others an effect of a medical condition without knowing what specifically to do about it. The feeling of isolation is a more dangerous factor impeding the health of an individual. Here are some of the reasons why interaction is beneficial to a person:

Better mental health

The more you interact with people, the more active your brain becomes. Most of the world-renown scholars and inventors came out with great exploits on account of the great interactions they had with people. You can never get ideas by just sitting alone with yourself. In fact, the process of knowledge dissemination entails that communication or dialogue is established between two or more persons. People who tend to stay isolated to themselves have more chances of making their brains more and more dormant. Sorrows and sad emotions are all evoked in your brain as you stay more secluded in interaction. Take, for example, children who are more actively involved with their peers eventually have higher intellectual capabilities.

Lower your risk of depression

Depression, as a.mental or emotional case, is mostly seen in people who have lower interaction with people. Although human relations isn't the only cause of depression, we find that a major control measure for handling depression is by engaging in friendly and uplifting conversations with people. You can be able to lighten the burdens that weigh you down as you communicate, laugh, smile and joke with others. Depression is a state of emotional sadness that thrives upon the lack of attention and moral support from persons around you and this is why patients suffering from such can opt to commit suicide.

One of the major factors attributed to cases of depression is loneliness. Depression has been found to be a contributory factor to the increase in young mortality facing the world today. You get to find so many people so sad and tired of living that they take their lives by their own hands. Depression can also be a source of stroke and increased heart rate variability. Sometimes as one gets more and more depressed, his adrenaline production begins to spike up, which could result in cardiac arrhythmia. Whatever the result, depression has been seen to have great implications on the health of an individual; this is why we must all do our best to reduce the number of cases we come up with.

Promotes a sense of safety, belonging and security

When persons suffer from insecurity and restlessness, it is mostly because they have no form of trust or security in the persons they have around. You would always feel not welcomed or unsafe when you keep on isolating yourself from others.

Allows you to confide in others and let them confide in you.

How can a person confide in you and share his or her experiences with you when you don't try to communicate with him/her. Good social interaction with people helps you understand and get to know them better.

Valtorta et all (2016) made serious attempts in trying to distinguish the effect of loneliness and social isolation on deaths associated with heart conditions. For his study, he implores information gathered from 11 cardiac cases and eight stroke cases. An increase in the heart condition was estimated at twenty-nine percent and another increase of thirty-two percent for stroke. This notable inflation in the figure also affected the recorded obesity and physical activity of people.

Solutions to social isolation

Many steps can be applied to cushion the effects of social isolation. At the top of this would be efforts made to spend time with people who help you manifest better habits, behaviors, nutrition and physical activity. It is only when you spend time with the right set of persons that you get to value the importance of social interaction. To be very careful in this, some relationships can lead to bad and poor habits like drinking, smoking, alcohol e.t.c, some friends and close allies can even introduce more emotional stress which should be avoided. When we put together all the negative effects of social interactions, we will still have the positive outcomes outweighing them. This means that no matter how lonely a person feels he should be, you still need the company of others to ensure that you live a fruitful life.

Sleep Disorders and Disruptive Cardiac Rhythm

The loss in the ability of a person to sleep well is what is termed as a sleep disorder. It can be caused by a number of factors, but at the top of the list is the inability of the vagal nerve to function properly. The vagal nerve is the connection link between the brain and the body which establishes rest and sleep. The inability of the brain to send signals and neurons across will hinder the ability of the person to sleep. Sleep disorders have become a common problem facing many across the world. Sleep disorders could also be attributed to stress.

Sources have it that in the U.S, a good number of people well above the third percentage of adults are able to sleep for about seven hours in a day. It was also discovered that a little above seventy percent of high school students are able to get eight hours of sleep daily.

Most of the time, when people experience sleep problems, it is caused by stress and over busy work schedules. Sleeping disorders become realistic when there are frequent challenges encountered while trying to sleep. This will invariably affect the entire health and progress of a person's daily life. With different types of sleep disorders, people have varying degrees of difficulty getting asleep. This is a factor hinged on whether they come back tired or not. For some people, the difficulty they experience doesn't go away even under extreme tiredness. This is why it is a huge challenge, imagine coming back from the office with all the workload and stress of the day, yet you still find it hard sleeping.

Sleeping difficulty could also be a result of some health challenges being experienced by the body. The problem will eventually go away once treatment is carried out for this kind of situation. In the event that the difficulty you experience while sleeping isn't caused by some medical issues, you will need to back up treatment with a change in your daily routines. You need to run a series of tests to determine the severity of the sleeping disorder you're dealing with before making conclusions. This will help you avoid the grave consequences that follow. You know that your ability to rest properly will always tell on your ability to be productive in your office or job. It will also lead to strains on your partners either in marriage or relationship. There are various types of sleeping disorders that have been identified, some caused by health challenges while others not. They include:

Insomnia

People suffering from this condition have difficulties sleeping, even when they do, they don't remain for long; there's always something cutting it short. It is mainly caused by stress, anxiety, hormonal problems. It can also be induced as a symptom of another medical condition. Insomnia leads to other issues like

- Depression
- Difficulty To Concentrate
- Irritability
- Weight Gain
- Reduced Work And School Performance

As bad as it is, we can find insomnia cases in about fifty percent of the population of the American adults who have either experienced it or are currently experiencing it. This condition can be found mostly in men and women. There are three-way insomnia can be classified.

- Chronic (this is when the condition has been constant for over a month)

- Intermittent (when it takes regular time cycles occurring)

- Transient (you could find this in persons who just have difficulties sleeping for some number of days at a time)

Sleep apnea

These conditions are characterized by brief pauses while sleeping. It is a serious issue, especially as it leads to shortages in the quantity of oxygen taken by the body. You would also experience this when you wake up regularly at night. It can occur in two ways, namely:

- Obstructive sleep apnea (here, the flow of air is obstructed because there is a limitation encountered as the air passes through the airways or because the airways have become narrow).

- Central sleep apnea (this typically happens when there is a breach in the connection between the brain and the muscles which aid breathing).

Parasomnias

This category of sleeping disorder is caused by movements and behaviors while sleeping. These behaviors include:

- Sleepwalking
- Sleep Talking

- Groaning
- Nightmares
- Bed Wetting
- Grinding and clenching of the tooth and jaw

Restless leg syndrome

Restless leg syndrome (RLS) is caused by a sensation in the legs. You will always experience this as a sensation, which is mostly present on your legs as you sleep. This isn't just limited to night experiences but also occurs during the day, although they happen most times at night. This difficulty is mostly attributed to other health conditions, which sometimes include Parkinson's disease. The exact cause is hard to determine.

Narcolepsy

These are sleep impulses experienced while the individual is still awake. Imagine you have to fall asleep without even knowing you just did until you wake up. This sometimes happens when you are tired and need rest. You can get into sleep paralysis, which means, you won't be able to love your kegs when you wake up. This condition may happen when you naturally are tired, but this happens more frequently In people with neurological disorders. If there is a problem with your brain and vagal nerve communication, you are prone to having this condition.

Symptoms of sleeping disorders

The symptoms experienced by many persons vary because the disorders are of varying degrees of severity. They may also be attributed to other health challenges. Here are some of the symptoms you are most likely to experience:

- Difficulty while falling and remaining asleep
- Fatigue during the day
- A sensation or impulse to sleep when it's not yet night
- Fluctuations in breathing pattern while sleeping
- An urge to move while falling asleep
- Changes to your sleep/wake schedule or time
- Irritability or anxiety
- Reduced performance at work or school
- Lack of concentration
- Depression
- Weight gain

Causes of sleep disorders

There are many health conditions that are responsible for disorders while sleeping. You still need to run a diagnosis to be certain if your challenge is a mental or a nervous issue. Examples of conditions that can cause a sleeping disorder are:

Allergies and respiratory problems

Allergies, cold, and infections on the respiratory system can alter breathing patterns when you sleep. When you are not able to breathe well, you will have difficulty sleeping.

Frequent urination

Urinating during night hours can cause a disruption in your sleep because your body gets so used to waking up to excrete urine. You might also have hormonal imbalances and urinary tract infections as another cause of sleep disorder. You should visit a doctor when you begin to notice signs of blood associated with your urine.

Chronic pain

When a person experiences pains, it makes it difficult to find sleep. You get to even wake up at moments or times when you never expected just because the pains are too much. Persons who have bone problems suffer this most of the time. This is why they are given sleeping and pain relief tablets so that they can sleep well. Some conditions that can result in pains are:

- Arthritis
- Chronic fatigue syndrome
- Fibro-myalgia
- Inflammatory bowel disease
- Persistent headaches
- Continuous lower back pain

When a person is stressed, you will naturally encounter difficulties while trying to sleep. You might even find yourself waking up at regular intervals. You might also be restless when you have a form of emotional pressure that keeps you all through the night thinking and meditating on thoughts. The negative effect of this is that when you don't get enough sleep, your body tends to run short on ideas for the next day. You will also experience tiredness and lag during the morning hours.

Chronic Inflammation

Inflammations are caused by processes that involve your body's defense to threats and signs of danger. These threats could be in the form of infections, injuries, or toxic substances being ingested into it. In the body's attempt to heal itself, it tries to release these substances out. Responses are triggered by your immune system to fight against these threats. Antibodies and some categories of proteins are also released into the bloodstream. The secretion of these antibodies and proteins are specifically to the damaged areas. The entire procedure is estimated to last for some hours or days (in the case of acute inflammation).

Chronic inflammations are formed when there is a delay in the response of the body in fighting foreign threats. This delay leaves your body in a state of alert. As time progresses, the negative effect of this condition will definitely affect your organs and tissue systems. Chronic inflammatory cases could also be the cause of a wider range of diseases, such as cancer and asthma.

Symptoms of chronic inflammation

Chronic inflammation or acute inflammation, as it is often called, has signs and symptoms which can be noticed on the physical body. These signs manifest as pains, swelling and coloration of body parts. The ease with which these signs manifest is such that they can be easily ignored; this makes it more deadly.

A crop section of other symptoms you would experience with chronic inflammation include:

- Fatigue
- Fever
- Mouth sores
- Rashes
- Abdominal pain
- Chest pain

These symptoms can be either less severe or extremely severe, depending on the duration in which the inflammation has lasted. In some cases, it could take months and years before you experience any sign.

Now lets carefully look at the different views on the manifestation of chronic inflammation.

- It could be an untreated form of an injury that has refused to heal, gradually decaying and accumulating dead cells.
- It also results from a disorder associated with the immune system where the antibodies released

attack tissues with no health condition, thus killing them. This occurs when there is misinformation in the cells to attack. Sometimes, the response can be linked to the failure of your vagus nerve to take necessary action being sent through from your brain.

- When you are exposed to long term industrious chemicals that are dangerous to your respiratory systems.

The causes of inflammation are not constant for every person. Some chronic inflammatory diseases don't have a specific cause attached to their formation. Through a series of researches, scientists have also identified other causes of chronic inflammation. These are listed below

- Smoking
- Obesity
- Alcohol consumption
- High levels of stress exposures

Effects of chronic inflammation on your body

It damages your cells and body tissues. When formed, chronic inflammation can alter your body's response in the secretion of antibodies. This releases them to the wrong location, thus affecting healthy cells, tissues and organs. Due to the failure of proper information on the area of attack, these antibodies gradually lead to further damages to the DNA, tissues and leave series of scars. As this continues, the general health of the body is destroyed, leading to other diseases.

- Cancer
- Heart disease
- Rheumatoid arthritis
- Type 2 diabetes
- Obesity
- Asthma
- Neurodegenerative diseases, such as Alzheimer's disease

Treatment of chronic inflammation

Since inflammation is caused by the body's default system in healing from threats, it is important that the systems that control such processes are kept in healthy conditions. One such system is the vagal nerve. This is why you need to always ensure that your vagal tone doesn't go below a healthy threshold. If for any reason, you notice that your vagal tone count is lower than expected, you should put steps in place to make sure that It is increased. In order to manage the longer-term implications of chronic inflammations, the following are advised.

Administration of drugs

Drugs like Nonsteroidal anti-inflammatory drugs (NSAIDs) are advised by your doctor to be taken as preventive measures. You can also be directed to pharmaceutical stores where you can get specific doses of aspirin, ibuprofen (Advil) and naproxen. All these drugs reduce the inflammatory formation and pains associated with it. Doctors also advise that these drugs be taken in recommended proportions to avoid other complications like peptic ulcer and kidney diseases.

The intake of steroids like corticosteroids helps boost the hormonal system. They help depress the immune system when they start attacking the healthy tissues and cells. As you use them consistently, you could develop vision problems, high blood pressure, and osteoporosis. You must ensure that the doses are prescribed by your doctor.

Intake of supplements

Some supplements are capable of reducing inflammations. These supplements come in the form of fish oils, lipoic acids, curcumin. These all have the potential of eliminating inflammations pertaining to cancer and heart diseases. There are spices that could be mixed to reduce chronic inflammatory diseases. Examples of such spices include ginger, garlic, and cayenne.

Dietary effects of chronic inflammation

The food you consume can have both negative and positive impacts on the formation of chronic inflammation.

Foods to eat

There are some types of foods you can eat that help prevent inflammations from forming. A variety of foods have anti-inflammatory properties. These include foods that are high in antioxidants and polyphenols, such as:

- Olive oil

- Leafy greens, such as kale and spinach
- Tomatoes
- Fatty fish, such as salmon, sardines, and mackerel
- Nuts
- Fruits, especially cherries, blueberries, and oranges

A good recommendation for diets that fight inflammation is the Mediterranean diet. This diet helps boost the body's ability to fight and defend against inflammations. There are certain foods you must also avoid as they have the potential of stirring up inflammatory responses in the body. They are mostly carbohydrates and chemically refined carbohydrate sources. Examples of these foods are;

- Refined carbohydrates, such as white bread and pastries
- Fried foods, such as french fries
- Red meat

In an attempt to be careful about what you eat, you find it completely hard taking these foods off from your diet, especially if you've been used to them. You don't necessarily have to get rid of them permanently. You can reduce the frequency with which you consume them.

Allowing inflammations will only leave you with more health conditions than you expect. You should seek out professional help in diagnosing your conditions through a series of tests and examinations. You should also endeavor to live healthy lifestyles by watching the classes of food you eat. The stimulation of the vagus nerve will help reduce your susceptibility to inflammatory conditions.

Dysfunctional Breathing

Disorders associated with breathing are commonly referred to as breathing pattern disorders. They are abnormal patterns experienced in respiratory processes. They are mostly related to breathing issues. They could be as small as upper chest breathing hyperventilation to more chronic cases of hyperventilation

They are chronic and reappearing changes to the breathing patterns of individuals. Although tied to some specific disease conditions, they are not solely caused by some respiratory infections. They don't manifest as diseases themselves but as alterations to the breathing pattern. This alteration is what hindered the smooth running of respiratory processes. They can be existing in partnership with other disease conditions.

Breathing pattern disorders are capable of causing damages to the mind, muscles, mood and general body metabolism rate. They can also be part of the reason why you develop chronic cases of fatigue, back, neck and pelvic pains, depression and anxiety. These disorders are influenced by the poor functioning of the vagal nerve system. Breathing coordination is brought about by a joint effort by the vagal nerve and other respiratory organs.

Clinically Relevant Anatomy

Our respiratory system begins in the thorax. The wall of this structure contains both the muscular and skeletal components of the breathing system. When we try to describe the respiratory system, we do so by classifying it into functional and anatomical parts. From the functional aspect of it, we have two divided zones. The first zone is called the conducting zone. This is located along with a connection from the nose to the bronchioles. It serves as a pathway for the movement of inhaled oxygen. The second zone is called the respiratory zone. This is mostly concerned with the exchange of the gases being inhaled. It is made up of the alveolar duct, the alveolar sac and the alveoli itself.

When we look into the anatomical divisions, we have the upper and lower respiratory tracts. The upper respiratory tract begins at the nose and terminates at the larynx. The lower respiratory tract begins at the trachea down to the alveoli.

An average of over ten percent of the total population has been diagnosed with hyperventilation syndrome. Some others have mild and serious levels of breathing disorders. Breathing disorders can be found in a higher percentage of the female gender, with an astonishing twelve percent difference with figures of the male gender. There have been little inputs to determine the extent of cases of dysfunctional breathing In children. Studies carried out reveals that only 5.3% of children have asthma and dysfunctional breathing. This is attributed to the poor control of the condition.

Disorders in breathing patterns occur when the ventilation received by the body exceeds the metabolic rate. This opens up to different symptoms and chemical changes. Sometimes failure in the ability of the upper chest to breathe properly will produce a shortage of carbon dioxide In the blood. The result of this process is respiratory diseases called alkaloid and even hypoxia or oxygen delivery to the tissues.

Breathing disorders have an effect on the biochemistry of the body and can cause alterations to the emotions, digestive functions, circulation and muscular structures involved in respiratory processes. Changes in the body's blood level, pH, pain threshold are also further effects of dysfunctional breathing patterns. Asides from being a disease condition, breathing disorders can produce some symptoms that look similar to those caused by infections and some health problems.

There are a lot of imbalances that occur on account of breathing disorders. They sometimes result from a previous condition that was not well attended to, thus causing a breathing disorder. The imbalances may manifest in the form of thoracic mobility, tension in respiratory muscles, chest wall movement disorders, and poor diaphragmatic descent.

Disorders experienced with breathing come in a different form for various individuals. Some conditions manifest in partnership with stress and anxiety, while others just affect the muscles and skeletal structures involved in breathing. There are identified symptoms that point to the presence of a breathing disorder; they include:

- Frequent sighing and yawning
- Breathing discomfort
- Disturbances while sleeping
- Erratic heartbeats
- Feeling of anxiety
- Pins and needle feelings around the body
- Upset gut/nausea
- Clammy hands
- Chest Pains
- Shattered confidence
- Being tired all the time
- Achy muscles and joints
- Dizzy spells or feeling spaced out
- Irritability or hypervigilance
- Feeling of 'air hunger'
- Breathing discomfort

Dysfunctional Digestive System

Disorders occurring in the digestive system include constipating, irritable bowel, hemorrhoids, fissures and so many more. These conditions can be prevented and reduced to a minimized rate by ensuring that a healthy lifestyle is maintained. Damages done to the vagal nerve or problems associated with the vagal nerve can give rise to such conditions. The vagal nerve is also connected to the digestive system and directly controls the movement of the stomach walls and intestines when food is being passed into it. When effective communication isn't established and movement isn't coordinated, the food wouldn't be digested as it needs to be. There are various types of disorders that could happen to the digestive (gastrointestinal) system, they include:

Functional gastrointestinal disorders

This type of disorder can make the gastrointestinal tract look okay and without any suspecting health issue. They are among the most popular conditions that could be associated with the gastrointestinal tract. Examples of this disorder include irritable bowel movement and constipation. There are several factors that could be responsible for obstructing the free movement of the internal organs. They are listed below.

Many factors may upset the GI (gastrointestinal) tract and its motility (or ability to keep moving). They include:

- Eating a diet low in fiber.
- Not enough exercise.
- Traveling or other changes in routine.
- Eating large amounts of dairy products.
- Stress.
- Resisting the urge to have a bowel movement.
- Resisting the urge to have bowel movements due to pain from hemorrhoids.
- Overusing laxatives (stool softeners) that, over time, weaken the bowel muscles.
- Taking antacid medicines containing calcium or aluminum.
- Taking certain medicines (especially antidepressants, iron pills, and strong pain medicines such as narcotics).
- Pregnancy.

Constipation

This is the inability of the bowel to pass out stool. This causes the excretion of stool reduced to thrice in a week; it may even occur incompletely when it is eventually passed out. It is caused by insufficient consumption of fibers and roughages in the food being consumed. The presence of these roughages enables the bowels to move smoothly and pass out the waste products. Constipation could also result from a change in the diet schedule being taken. When bowel movement occurs, it is usually accompanied with pains in an individual when he/she suffers from constipation. You may also encounter difficulty while passing stool and this would cause other anal problems like fissures and hemorrhoids. Constipation is not so much of a critical health challenge.

The treatment of constipation can be achieved by applying the following medical procedures:

- Increasing the amount of fiber you eat.
- Exercising regularly.
- Moving your bowels when you have the urge (resisting the urge causes constipation).

If these treatments don't work, you can also add laxatives as a form of temporal solution. You should endeavor not to take them without prescription or in excess so that it doesn't increase the severity of the condition. You must take laxatives according to the prescription of your doctor or pharmacist.

Irritable bowel syndrome (IBS)

This can also be called (spastic colon); it is a digestive system disease where the muscles in the colon are forced to contract more than they should. They can be triggered by drugs, emotional stress and anxiety. Some symptoms that show that one is suffering from Irritable bowel syndrome are:

- Abdominal pain and cramps.
- Excess gas.
- Bloating.
- Change in bowel habits such as harder, looser, or more urgent stools than normal.
- Alternating constipation and diarrhea.

The various ways it can be treated are;

- Avoiding caffeine.
- Increasing fiber in the diet.

- Monitoring which foods trigger IBS (and avoiding these foods).
- Minimizing stress or learning different ways to cope with stress.
- Sometimes taking medicines as prescribed by your healthcare provider.

Structural gastrointestinal disorders

These kinds of disorders to the gastrointestinal system are abnormal and cause the digestive system to malfunction. You might need to carry out surgical procedures to get these conditions removed. Some examples of these disorders include hemorrhoids, colon polyps, cancer, inflammatory bowel disease.

Colitis

Colitis is a medical condition that results in the inflammation of the bowels. It could be in various forms and classes.

- Infectious colitis.
- Ulcerative colitis (cause is unknown).
- Crohn's disease (cause is unknown).

- Ischemic colitis (caused by not enough blood going to the colon).
- Radiation colitis (resulting from radiotherapy).

Colitis produces other symptoms like rectal bleeding, abdominal cramps and urgency (frequent and immediate need to empty the bowels). Treatment depends on the diagnosis, which is made by colonoscopy and biopsy.

Dysfunctional Heart Rate

The heart squeezes and relaxes each time it beats. The squeezing of the heart muscles along the cycle is called systole. The relaxation of the muscles is called diastole. When the ventricles (the heart's major pumping chambers) squeeze, they push blood out of the heart and into the blood vessels. After the ventricles have finished squeezing, they relax. This allows them to refill with blood to get ready to squeeze again.

The heart muscles are flexible enough to be stiffened when there are malfunctioning in the signals being sent to it. The contraction and relaxation of the heart are aided by the autonomic control of the nervous system. If this control isn't exercised properly, there might be complications while trying to relax itself. When this happens, the ventricles have a harder time relaxing themselves. As the blood being pumped increases in pressure, the blood being released can flow into the lungs through the blood vessel. Dysfunction in the heart rate can also result in shortages while breathing, a medical term referred to a diastolic heart failure.

Causes of dysfunctional heart rate:

The following factors are responsible for dysfunctional heart rate:

- High blood pressure
- Hypertrophic cardiomyopathy (the walls of the heart become thick and stiff)
- Aortic stenosis (narrowing in one of the heart valves)
- Coronary artery disease
- Restrictive cardiomyopathy (scars or deposits that make the heart muscle stiff)
- Aging

This medical condition is a common challenge facing many aged adults. This happens because as persons grow older, the coordination of involuntary activities reduces. Sometimes the dysfunction may result in more severe conditions of heart failure

Symptoms of heart dysfunction

There is no know obvious symptoms you could use to identify when you are faced with this condition. Most of all the symptoms you would experience would be centered around your heart rate and difficulty in breathing

Shortness of breath or trouble breathing:

People with heart dysfunction have trouble while carrying out exercises because they run short of breath more often. You might also find them waking up periodically at night due to the struggles they encounter with breathing while sleeping. People like this are unable to lie on their backs because when they do, it makes it difficult for them to breathe properly.

Fast or irregular heartbeat:

Due to the fluctuations in the contraction and relaxation of the heart, you will discover that the pace with which the heart pumps blood will be unstable. This is why you can have a series of irregular palpitations.

Diagnosis of heart dysfunction

You will need to consult medical help for advice and a series of tests carried out to determine the severity of your condition. Your medical doctor would also advise on the necessary steps to take in order to ensure that your vagal tone doesn't triple too low.

The series of test carried out include:

Chest X-ray

The use of an Echocardiogram (ECK) to measure and record heart rate. The Echocardiogram makes use of ultrasonic waves to determine the rate at which your blood is pumped.

Treatment

The basic thing to do while trying to deal with any disease condition is to identify the root cause. When the root cause has been identified, we can know what steps to take. When dealing with dysfunctional heart rates, we acknowledge that for worse case scenarios, we might have to carry out surgical procedures or recommend healthy eating habits and lifestyle.

You will probably need to take medicines your health care provider will prescribe.

Chapter 4

Substances That May Affect Your Vagus Nerve

The vagal nerve is one of the most important cranial nerve systems in the body. It must be protected from any form of harm or danger. Any impact or defect in the effective communication between the vagal nerve and the brain can result in deadly health challenges. Since the vagal nerve is in charge of monitoring and maintaining constant heart rate, digestion, and reduction in stress levels, we must be careful of things and activities that hamper its safety. There are certain substances you take that can be harmful to the vagal nerve. It is important we take a look at these substances.

Botox

Botox is a drug mainly injected into the body. It is composed of the botulinum toxin type A chemical. It is produced by a bacteria specifically for the relaxation of muscles. It sometimes is mistaken for the same toxin that causes food poisoning. The dosage a person is given would determine the kind of effect to be experienced. The doses are meant to be given in small quantities.

When this injection is administered, it goes directly to the muscles and nerves with the aim of obstructing any communication. This process is what brings about the relaxation of the muscles. The bad part of this is that it can also block communication between your brain and some essential muscles by affecting the vagal nerve. This could lead to more severe complications.

A lot of people keep on asking if it's safe to take botox, medically we advise that whatever the need be to consume botox, you do so in small quantities as prescribed by a medical practitioner. It is only when this is done that botox becomes safe.

Botox not only finds its application in the medical world but also in the cosmetic industry. Some cosmetic brands and companies introduce little amounts of botox into their formulas for some treatment purposes. These applications do not bring as much consequence as those of the injection. The ability of the drug to reduce wrinkles and lining on the skin has made it a good option for many fashion brands.

It can also cause relaxation to the muscles that are responsible for crow's feet, wrinkling on the eyes and eyebrows. The following are muscle conditions botox is used to treat:

- Lazy eye
- Eye twitching
- Chronic migraines
- Neck spasms (cervical dystonia)
- Overactive bladder
- Excessive sweating (hyperhidrosis)
- Certain neurological conditions, such as cerebral palsy

Whatever this need be for the administration of botox, you must also consider its long term and short term side effects, especially as it affects your vagal nerve. Common symptoms to notice when botox injections are given are:

- Pain, swelling, or bruising at the injection site
- Headache
- Fever
- Chills

You would want to avoid a whole lot of eye complications even as you opt for botox injections given as a prescription for eye conditions. A few of such complications include

- Drooping eyelids
- Uneven eyebrows
- Dry eyes
- Excessive tearing

Certain Antibiotics

Antibiotics have been discovered to have an effect on the immune system by affecting the production of antibodies and antigens that fight germs, infections and diseases. Although not all antibiotics are capable of causing such, we must be careful of the type of antibiotic consumed. Antibiotics are taken to boost the body's immune system against any form of external threats. Some antibiotics have an adverse effect on some individuals, while some others don't. The nervous transfer that occurs from the vagal nerve is what is being interfered with and obstructed.

Some studies have been carried out to understand why the reaction varies in different individuals. The damages caused by antibiotics can be as serious as resulting in memory loss, retardation and death of brain cells.

As useful as antibiotics can be, there is still a need to make a careful examination of what category of antibiotics is being administered. When applied in the wrong doses and medical conditions, they do much more than helping to fight disease-causing organisms. Some antibiotics are capable of causing damages to the digestive system by attacking the walls of the stomach and intestinal movement areas.

Some of the gut-related problems have also been traced back to the wrong consumption of antibiotics. They find their way into the gut killing all the microbes, either good or bad and leaving worse scars behind. Every person has a unique chemical composition. This is why tests need to be carried.

Antibiotics is a way of inhibiting the vagal nerve result and it causes peripheral neuropathy. It is a health condition where you experience pains and feelings of tingling, just like what you experience when you have a set of needles being pierced into your hands, arms, legs and foot. Antibiotics could also initiate weakness of the body muscles and a kind of loss in the sensations on some body parts. The damages to the vagal nerve could as well be made permanent. You may think that by ending the dosages of the antibiotics, you will eliminate the side effects and discontinue them from manifesting. This is why you need to be well informed of the effects of the antibiotic you are about to take before you do to avoid permanent damages to your vagal nerve.

Heavy Metals

Heavy metals are chemical materials that can be found in deposits that occur naturally. They find their applications in our day to day activities like medicine, industry, and agriculture. Heavy metals are of different types and varying compositions. The body requires, to some extent, the presence of these metals. When the proportion of the metals available exceeds its allowable limit, the body begins to react.

The intake of food and supplements that have high concentrations of heavy metals should be discouraged. This is because they affect the vagus nerve. As they continue to accumulate in the bloodstream, they begin to disrupt the smooth functioning of the vagus nerve. Most of the effects of heavy metals can only be possible when the vagus nerve is not well protected. The following are examples of heavy metals that, in larger quantities, can be disastrous to the human body.

- Mercury
- Lead
- Cadmium

- Arsenic

The body naturally contains other metals like zinc, iron, and copper. These are available in specified proportions to enable the body to carry out some bodily functions. Their presence in the body is not toxic alone. When the amounts and proportion of these metals exceed the allowable limit, they become dangerous. The soft tissues of the body are capable of absorbing these metals when present in large quantities.

Apart from exposures from food, these metals can also be introduced into the body through air, water consumption, medicines, industrial and painting operations. Some drugs contain some amount of heavy metals. These drugs need to be prohibited since not everyone reacts to them in the same way. The poisoning associated with heavy metals is quite not common, especially in the U.S. The type of exposure and the level to which the metals are accumulated will determine the effect the individual experiences. There are chemicals the body secretes to detoxify the amount of heavy metals deposited. The following are the symptoms individuals face, which point towards heavy metal accumulation. The symptoms can be varied for different individuals, but there are general symptoms that can be common to almost everyone.

Common symptoms across several types of heavy metal poisoning include:

- Diarrhea
- Nausea
- Abdominal pain
- Vomiting
- Shortness of breath
- Tingling in your hands and feet
- Chills
- Weakness

The formation of weaknesses in children is attributed to the accumulation of heavy metals in the body. Heavy metals are part of the nutrients needed to keep the baby and avoid miscarriages. There are some other types of symptoms that are specifically tied to the presence of certain heavy metals. For example, when iron is in excess, the symptoms that will be experienced would be different from that of arsenic.

Examples of mercury poisoning symptoms:

- Lack of coordination

- Muscle weakness
- Hearing and speech difficulties
- Nerve damage in your hands and face
- Vision changes
- Trouble walking

Examples of lead poisoning symptoms:

- Constipation
- Aggressive behavior
- Sleep problems
- Irritability
- High blood pressure
- Loss of appetite
- Anemia
- Headaches
- Fatigue
- Memory loss
- Loss of developmental skills in children

Excessive Sugar Intake

One of the consequences of having to take in much amount of sugar is the possibility of sending the body into a state of diabetes. This is not merely sponsored by the intake of sugar but by the inability of the insulin being produced by the body to convert all the sugars.

The vagal nerve is responsible for the control of the secretion of insulin in the body. As part of its digestive roles, the vagal nerve enables the right amount of insulin is produced. When the consumption of sugar becomes too much, it affects the rate at which insulin is produced and thus leading to the inability of the insulin being produced to carryout conversion. The body doesn't need sugars; that why it must be converted into glucose or, at other times, stored as excess fat.

A research was conducted with the aim to identify how the vagus nerve essentially affects the digestion of glucose in the body. The outcome showed that whenever the body took in carbohydrate food, a signal was sent from the brain through the vagal nerve to commence the production of insulin. Since the vagus nerve is connected to virtually almost every part of the body, it controls most of the essential processes. Imagine eating food and in the process of eating, you discover that the food you ate last night had not been digested due to the inability of the vagal nerve to relay hormones that should kick start the process of digestion. This is what happens when you increase your sugar intake beyond what is recommended. Diabetic conditions are the result of stress and pressure placed in your body to produce insulin. You should know that the older you get, the more difficult it is for some of your systems and organs to regulate themselves. Thus it is advisable for us to reduce the kind of foods we eat, especially those that have excessive sugar components.

When the vagal nerve is stimulated, it becomes more effective at releasing hormones and impulses that aid in the digestion of sugars. Taking in so much amount of sugar affects the role the vagus nerve plays in the gastrointestinal processes. Glucose homeostasis is the process involved in the metabolism of carbohydrates to glucose. This can only be achieved by the constant secretion of insulin aided by the vagal nerve. As part of preventive ways for the creation of diabetic conditions, people are advised to be more watchful of the diets they consume. A food nutritionist or dietician should be able to advise you on the type of meal to eat, especially if you have a low insulin production rate.

The consumption of sugary foods also affects the movement of food down the esophagus, a rare condition experienced by a few. This medical condition is called swallow syncope. It results from the loss of consciousness due to a reflex action from the brain to the esophagus.

The end... almost!

Hey! We've made it to the final chapter of this book, and I hope you've enjoyed it so far.

If you have not done so yet, I would be incredibly thankful if you could take just a minute to leave a quick review on the product page of this book from where the purchase was made, even if it is a few sentences!

Reviews are not easy to come by, and as an independent author with a little marketing budget, I rely on you, my readers, to leave a short review on my book.

Even if it is just a sentence or two!

So if you really enjoyed this book, please...

>> Leave a short review on the product page of this book from where the purchase was made, even if it is a few sentences!

I truly appreciate your effort to leave your review, as it truly makes a huge difference.

Chapter 5

Stimulating Your Vagus Nerve

We have in previous chapters, talked about the effect and dangers of having a malfunctioning vagus nerve. In light of this, the vagus nerve must thus be activated to function properly and effectively. This can be achieved through various activities and procedures. In this chapter, we will be taking a closer look at the activities that can be done to improve the state of the vagal nerve, some of which we had previously touched on.

Natural Exercises and Practices

Deep and slow breathing

Since the vagal nerve is controlled by a set of parasympathetic nervous impulses, better control and coordination of this nerve is possible. This can be done by practicing deep and slow breathing techniques. As earlier discussed, most people breathe through the lungs (chest area) instead of the diaphragm. In this section, I would describe how to breathe properly using the deep and slow diaphragmatic breathing technique. This can be very useful when the body is going through a state of anxiety and stress. You can take some minutes, deliberately lower the speed at which you take in air. The inhalation and exhalation of air are done from the diaphragm. You should be able to notice your stomach move upwards and downwards. Doing this over time will stimulate your vagal nerve. The essence of this is to enhance the speed with which your vagal nerve sends impulses to your brain and back to the various sections of your body.

To start breathing from your diaphragm, do the following:

- Sit either on a chair while resting your head, neck, and shoulders against the back of the chair or lay your back against the floor or bed, aided by a pillow to your head and feet.

- Lay one of your hand on your upper chest and the other on your belly.

- Shut your eyes and breathe in deeply and slowly into your belly via your nose (i.e., to expand your diaphragm) to the count of five, take a pause then

- Slowly exhale through your mouth to the count of ten

- Repeat the same process for about 5-10 minutes

Humming, Chanting and Singing

In the previous chapters, I explained how the vagal nerve actually runs down to the connection of your vocal cords. They are also linked to the muscles at the back of your throat. When you hum or sing, air flows down to your local folds, causing a vibration. This vibration is what produces the audible sounds produced from the mouth. As a form of stress relief therapy, doctors advise that you sing and make melodies with your mouth when you feel you're gradually getting depressed, anxious or tensed. This works because as the vagal folds vibrate alongside the muscles, they equally cause a vibration of the vagal nerve. This vibration helps it receive and return signal as it should. Think of it like a metal whose vibration affects another close metal and brings both of them into a mutual vibration. Humming and singing have also been proven to aid in the stabilization of the heart rate and improve the vagal tone value.

Humor Therapy

Humour is a very good relaxation therapy for the body. When you stay happy, you increase your lifespan by a little percentage. Humour therapy involves you occasionally being around friends and people who can evoke smiles and laughter on your face. A reason why many come down with stress of varying degrees is that they don't take out time to laugh, smile and enjoy the beauty of life. You can't get more out of life when you don't laugh and smile. When you are happy, you indirectly prime positive reactions of people to you. It could be a warm greeting, an act of kindness, e.t.c. Studies show that when a person smiles, their brain becomes more productive and their mental power is heightened.

When you see employees who are always joyful and happy, you would observe that they have higher productive rates and better health conditions. This is true for so many reasons, some being that the brain works by firing thousands and millions of neural receptors. These neural receptors enable the part of the brain responsible for intellect to function properly. When you smile and laugh, you relax the brain muscles and enable more signals to be sent across it. When you regularly practice humor therapy, you will discover that your vagal tone will always be at an appropriate condition and not fall below healthy thresholds.

Gargling

Gargling produces the same effect as humming and singing. Little children love to do this and most adults don't understand the importance of this. We tend to shut them up and discourage them. Gargling is a very effective way of stimulating the vagal nerve. Why is this so? It aids in the vibration of the vocal folds and muscles, which also have an effect on the vagal nerve.

When you want to gargle, place an amount of water inside your mouth (a safe amount you can swallow without spilling). Make sure that your head is slightly tilted upwards to enable the water to stay in your mouth while you slide it open. With this done, you vibrate the water contained in your mouth by vibrating your vocal muscles. It looks more like trying to make sounds while the water still remains in your mouth. If you do this effectively, you should be making a childish sound just like the sounds children make when they brush their teeth. As you do this repeatedly for a couple of minutes, your vagal nerve becomes stimulated.

You can also carry out this exercise as a form of relaxation. The mere thought of you carrying out this exercise is relaxing. As you gargle with the water in your mouth, take your mind off every and any thoughts you have on your mind. You would find yourself more relieved than you expected. As your vocal folds begin to vibrate, they send waves down the vagus nerve and back. This constant activity wakes up every dormant area of the nerve. Since the nerve comprises a long connection of neurons, it is possible that some certain areas of the nerve endings have become dormant and cold. The waves sent through the vibration helps to reawaken every part of the connection.

Exposure to Cold

Exposures to cold is another effective way of improving and stimulating the vagal nerve. Cold water has a lot of advantages and benefits to the human body. Cold water therapies are known for their ability to help you prolong your reaction to times of shock and stress while triggering the flight and fight hormones. These triggers are most useful when faced with some sort of danger or having to deal with a kind of stress. In order to make sure that these events don't break you down or send you into a state of heart failure, you must prepare your response system to deal with them.

The effects of cold water on the vagal nerve also go far as affecting the immune system. There have been varying degrees of studies carried out to see the connection between cold water and the immune system. These studies have shown that the immune system can be enhanced by exposing the body to cold water. The experiment was done on some persons who volunteered. They wanted to know how to control their nervous reactions.

It is a known fact that the involuntary responses of the body can not be controlled. Some of these involuntary responses include breathing, heartbeat, secretion of hormones and a whole lot more. We have seen this control already achieved by people who spend time meditating and attending yoga lessons. They have, over time, come to learn how to bring the body into total control where each response to a stimulus is self-determined. Science took a backlog on this method but later came up with concrete findings on how these actions are possible.

We have now understood that the immune system has a connection with cold water exposures. The series of activities that involve soaking the body in a bathtub or container filled with water reduces irregular breathing patterns. As you continue to practice this, you will have heightened your vagal time response.

Yoga

There is a connection between yoga and the stimulation of the vagus nerve. Yoga helps in strengthening the body's relaxation mechanism by reducing blood pressure, improving breathing and creating better activity around the nervous system. Students of yoga classes all have better and improved stress handling and metabolic rates. This is possible because yoga focuses on the parasympathetic nervous activities. Regular yoga lessons can lessen your depression risks by 80%. Mood complexities and anxiety issues can also be dealt with through yoga exercises. Yoga supports mental health and brings a balance to the vagus nerve network. More and more people are becoming aware of its benefits to the well-being of an individual. This has caused an increase in the number of yoga classes and centers. The number of students applying for yoga sessions continues to double as it is now a cheap method of managing the nervous system. As you practice yoga, one effect you would be looking out for is better control over your body system. This is guaranteed through the effect it has on your vagus nerve.

Meditation

Meditation is the ability of the brain/mind to lose focus of surrounding thoughts and worries and focus on a particular thought or idea. This can be achieved through a number of ways. Since it entails personal efforts, there are a countless number of ways people practice this. Meditation is becoming a widely accepted stress-relieving technique for many persons. This is because meditation works on soothing the nerves and nervous responses. Through a series of research, scientists have come to discover that persons who meditate more often have heightened vagal tones and great ability to manage their thoughts and stress. Meditation also focuses on your breathing patterns to bring it to a slow, consistent, and peaceful pace. Mediation acts like a fast therapy for overcoming anxiety and depression because it improves your mood and healthy structure of the vagal nerve

Massage

Through scientific research, it is discovered that massaging stimulates and increases the activity that goes on in the vagal nerve. There are areas of the body that can be massaged to achieve the desired result. One of such parts would be to massage the foot. This helps to bring relief to the nerves and increase the heart's variability. This is why many people prefer to be given a foot massage when experiencing some form of tension or stress. The areas around the throat can also be massaged to stimulate the vagus nerve. This reduces the occurrence of heart seizures and brings better communication between the brain and the vagus nerve. It is more advisable to go for massages at least once a month.

Movement or Exercise

Health experts have discovered that exercises have a way of stimulating your vagus nerve by increasing your heart rate and, by so doing, improves your parasympathetic activity, as well as training your body to easily recover from stress.

Asides the many effects of exercises on the health of the body, the help it renders in the development of a healthy brain and mind is one advantage we cannot overlook. On account of this, you should try your best to exercise regularly at least once every day. If your routine is too busy to accommodate such, you could fall back on an average of 4 times a week. When you exercise, you open up your sweat pores, which allow for the release of waste in the form of sweat. As you do this consistently, you would notice an increase in your body's nervous system. It is more advisable to stick to routine exercises you're more comfortable with. Examples of exercises you could practice include sprinting, walking, and weight lifting.

Food and Dietary Supplement

Probiotics

Probiotics are live microorganisms (usually bacteria) that can be found in food or supplement and are intended to reproduce, maintain and or improve the healthiness of the good bacteria in our body such as that found in our gut.

There have been astonishing discoveries pertaining to the relationship between bacteria in the gut and the vagus nerve. Research has shown that these bacteria improve brain function when the vagus nerve is impacted. These bacteria modify the receptors responsible for the secretion of stress hormones, depression and anxiety. This makes them able to lower the response time the body uses when it engages in stress and unnecessary worries. The communication and flow of neurons between the gut and the brain is aided by the vagus nerve.

When the gut microbiome is overrun by pathogenic (bad) bacteria, the result is the creation of the breeding ground for inflammation. Probiotics help the vagus nerve to fight off inflammation.

Lactobacillus Rhamnosus and Bifidobacterium Longum are the two main species most probiotic supplements are made of. Also, fermented foods such as yogurt, kefir, kimchi, sauerkraut, sauerkraut, cheese, kombucha, and miso are known to be rich in probiotics. So, you may want to make these foods a part of your diet.

Omega-3 Fatty Acids

These class of acids is very vital to your body for a lot of reasons. They are part of the essential minerals, which unfortunately cannot be produced by your body. They must be consumed from external sources. The best sources of these acids are salmon fish, walnuts, flaxseed, soybean oil, and seaweed. They improve the efficient functioning of your nervous system by stimulating your vagus nerve.

Omega 3 fatty acid-rich foods, when taken, works on the nervous impulses so that you can exercise more control over your mental system. Sometimes with addictions, you might not be in control over the situation because your control over your parasympathetic nervous system is weak. Omega 3 fatty acid-rich foods help to breach this gap.

They not only help turn on your parasympathetic mode, thereby increasing your vagal tone and activity, they also help to overcome habits and addictions. The next time you see someone struggling genuinely from an addiction e.g., smoking, alcohol consumption, omega 3 fatty acid-rich foods, especially salmon fish, can be recommended for consumption.

When there are a high amount of omega 3 fatty acid-rich foods in your body system, you will live free from high blood pressure conditions and heart rate imbalance issues. Omega 3 fatty acids not only help prevent damages to the vagus nerve, they also quicken the healing processes for injuries sustained to the nerves in general.

Eicosapentaenoic acid (EPA) and Docosahexaenoic acid (DHA) are the two main types of omega- 3 fatty acids. Fish diets that are rich in DHA and EPA are salmon, mackerel, shrimp, seabass, oysters, and sardines, while seaweed and algae are vegetable diets that also contain DHA and EPA.

Passive Methods of Stimulation

Auricular Acupuncture

Auricular acupuncture is a type of therapy that has to do with the opening of the passageways where signals and neurons are sent from the heart to the vagus nerve and vice versa by providing a medium of stimulation via the ear. The points (insertion of needles into specific points on the ear) at which the acupunctures are made are the pathways through which the signals travel/move to the vagus nerve. The signals essentially need to be relayed to the brain through the vagus nerve. The acupuncture aids the signals to get to the vagus nerve faster and more adequately. The benefit of having this type of therapy is that it not only increases vagal activity and tone, nor provides more room for the vagus nerve to regulate and control the formation of inflammation in the organs of the body, but also, it helps in the treatment of depression, anxiety, epilepsy, and digestive disorders according to research.

Electrical Stimulation

This invokes the stimulation of the vagus nerve by the implantation of a clinical device on the chest, which sends electrical impulses to the brain. This device has been certified as an acceptable method by the FDA as a remedy to nerval imbalances, including seizures and depression.

This device is implanted in the body through surgical procedures just below the skin on the chest, where it is connected to the vagus nerve on the left side of the body. When the device is turned on, electrical signals are sent across the vagus nerve to the brain.

In recent times, new technologies have been introduced that are not invasive (not requiring surgical implantation). These new stimulating devices are also effective for the stimulation of the vagus nerve as they bring reliefs from depression, varying levels of stress, anxiety and other conditions associated with nerval disorders. Some of these new technologies are the gammaCore, which the FDA has approved its use in the US, and has also been cleared for use in Europe. Another of such devices is the NEMOS system, a device which when applied to the ear, stimulates the vagus nerve.

A greater percentage of people living with epilepsy do not respond to other stimulation methods. This option (electrical stimulation) reduces the occurrence of seizures and other complications associated with a low vagal tone. Likewise, when individuals have tried taking prescribed medications to suppress depression, anxiety and stress without any changes, they could opt for this stimulation method.

Conclusion

Exercising control over the nervous system seems to be a big deal for many people. This has led to frustration when faced with challenges like stress, anxiety, depression and so on, and has unfortunately for many, led to their untimely death.

To be able to stimulate the vagus nerve to function properly, you need to take a look at its structure, anatomy and its general functions. This will arm you with adequate knowledge on how best to get this nerve to work optimally.

With the points discussed in this book, you now better understand the different health conditions that can result when the vagus nerve is damaged and why you should be careful of the food and substances allowed into your body. Above all, with the methods of stimulation discussed in the pages of this book, you are now equipped to taking charge of your health and wellbeing for good by practicing any of the methods that are comfortable for you, depending on your current health situation.

Finally, I urge you to take personal responsibility for your health by making the tips shared in this book become a part of your daily life routine.

References

Seladi-Schulman, J. (2018, July 31). *Vagus Nerve Overview*. Healthline. https://www.healthline.com/human-body-maps/vagus-nerve#problems

Yazdi, P. (2020, January 6). *19 Factors That May Stimulate Your Vagus Nerve Naturally*. SelfHacked. https://selfhacked.com/blog/32-ways-to-stimulate-your-vagus-nerve-and-all-you-need-to-know-about-it/

Calming your nerves and your heart through meditation. (2014, January 9). Science in the News. http://sitn.hms.harvard.edu/flash/2009/issue61/

Caffrey, J. (2019, November 18). *How to access the Vagus nerve. Parasympathetic State via cold water.* Justin Caffrey - The Master of Mindset. https://www.justincaffrey.com/my-blog/2019/3/6/cold-water-and-the-vagus-nerve

Cohen, M. R. (2013, September 3). *New warnings for common antibiotic class.*

Https://Www.Inquirer.Com.
https://www.inquirer.com/philly/blogs/healthcare
/New-warnings-for-common-antibiotic-class.html

4 reasons behind an irregular heartbeat. (2018, February 9).
Geisinger. https://www.geisinger.org/health-and-
wellness/wellness-articles/2018/02/09/16/06/4-
reasons-behind-an-irregular-heartbeat

Brown, S. (2018, February 13). *Is It PTSD, Depression, or
Both?* WebMD.
https://www.webmd.com/depression/depression-
ptsd-vs-depression

Vagus nerve. (2020, August 17). Kenhub.
https://www.kenhub.com/en/library/anatomy/the
-vagus-nerve

*The vagus nerve and the inflammatory reflex—linking
immunity and metabolism.* (2012, December 1).
PubMed Central (PMC).
https://www.ncbi.nlm.nih.gov/pmc/articles/PMC
4082307/

Lightning Source UK Ltd.
Milton Keynes UK
UKHW022121300522
403744UK00004B/496